The Best Dash Diet Cookbook

Quick, Easy and Delicious Recipes and Meals for Everyday Tasty Recipes with Low Sodium Dishes to Lower your Blood Pressure.

Terry Donovan

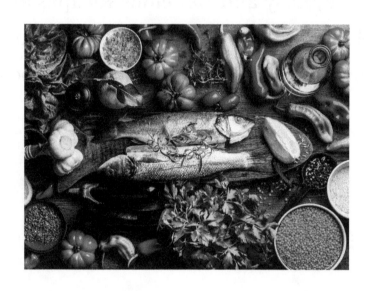

Table of Contents

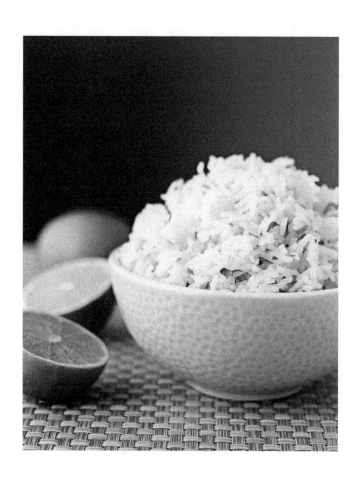

Lemon Salmon with Kaffir Lime

Preparation time: 15 minutes

Cooking time: 30 minutes

Servings: 8

Ingredients:

- A whole side of salmon fillet

- 1 thinly sliced lemon

- 2 kaffir torn lime leaves

- 1 quartered and bruised lemongrass stalk

- 1 ½ cups fresh coriander leaves

Directions:

1. Warm-up oven to 350 F. Covers a baking pan with foil sheets, overlapping the sides (enough to fold over the fish).

2. Put the salmon on the foil, top with the lemon, lime leaves, the lemongrass, and 1 cup of the coriander leaves. Option: season with salt and pepper.

3. Bring the long side of the foil to the center before folding the seal. Roll the ends to close up the salmon. Bake for 30 minutes. Transfer the cooked fish to a platter. Top with fresh coriander. Serve with white or brown rice.

Nutrition:

Calories 103

Protein 18g

Carbohydrates 43.5g

Fat 11.8g

Sodium 170mg

Baked Fish Served with Vegetables

Preparation time: 15 minutes

Cooking time: 30 minutes

Servings: 4

Ingredients:

- 4 haddock or cod fillets, skinless

- 2 Zucchinis, sliced into thick pieces

- 2 red onions, sliced into thick pieces

- 3 large tomatoes, cut in wedges

- ¼ cup black olives pitted

- ¼ cup flavorless oil (olive, canola, or sunflower)

- 1 Tablespoon lemon juice

- 1 Tablespoon Dijon mustard

- 2 garlic cloves, minced

- Salt and pepper to season

- ½ cup chopped parsley

Directions:

1. Warm oven to 400 F. In a large baking dish, drizzle some oil over the bottom. Place the fish in the middle. Surround the fish with the zucchini, tomato,

onion, and olives. Drizzle more oil over the vegetables and fish. Season with salt and pepper.

2. Place the baking dish in the oven. Bake within 30 minutes, or until the fish is flaky and vegetables are tender. In another bowl, whisk the lemon juice, garlic, mustard, and remaining oil. Set aside.

3. Split the cooked vegetables onto plates, then top with the fish. Drizzle the dressing over the vegetables, fish. Garnish with parsley.

Nutrition:

Calories 91

Protein 18.7g

Carbohydrates 41g

Fat 7.6g

Sodium 199mg

Fish in A Vegetable Patch

Preparation time: 15 minutes

Cooking time: 20 minutes

Servings: 3

Ingredients:

- 1-pound halibut fillet, skinless

- 1 Tablespoon flavorless oil (olive, canola, or sunflower)

- 1 cup tomato sauce

- 1 ½ Tablespoons Worcestershire sauce

- 2 large lemons, juiced

- 1 celery stick, diced

- ½ green pepper, chopped

- 1 large carrot, diced

- ½ an onion, diced

- 1 lemon, sliced

Directions:

1. Warm oven to 400 F. In a small saucepan, combine the tomato sauce, Worcestershire sauce, and lemon juice. Heat for 5 minutes.

2. In a shallow baking dish, drizzle oil along the bottom. Place the vegetables along the bottom and lay the fish over the vegetables. Pour the sauce over the fish. Cover with foil.

3. Bake fillet for 15 minutes, or until the fish is cooked and flaky. Dish out the vegetables, place the fish over the top. Garnish the fish with the lemon slices. Serve with white or brown rice.

Nutrition:

Calories 80

Protein 18.9g

Carbohydrates 62g

Fat 9g

Sodium 276mg

Spicy Cod

Preparation time: 15 minutes

Cooking time: 30 minutes

Servings: 4

Ingredients:

- 2 pounds cod fillets

- 1 Tablespoon flavorless oil (olive, canola, or sunflower)

- 2 cups low sodium salsa

- 2 tablespoons fresh chopped parsley

Directions:

1. Warm oven to 350 F. In a large, deep baking dish, drizzle the oil along the bottom. Place the cod fillets in the dish. Pour the salsa over the fish.

2. Cover with foil for 20 minutes. Remove the foil last 10 minutes of cooking. Bake in the oven for 20 – 30 minutes, until the fish is flaky. Serve with white or brown rice. Garnish with parsley.

Nutrition:

Calories 110

Protein 16.5g

Carbohydrates 83g

Fat 11g

Sodium 186mg

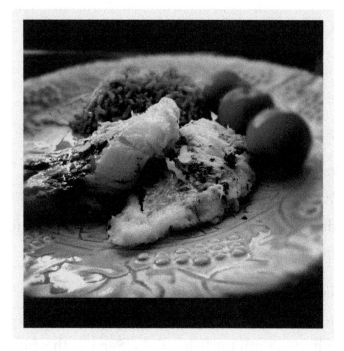

Easy Shrimp

Preparation time: 15 minutes

Cooking time: 10 minutes

Servings: 4

Ingredients:

- 1-pound cooked shrimp

- 1 pack mixed frozen vegetables

- 1 garlic clove, minced

- 1 teaspoon butter or margarine

- ¼ cup of water

- 1 package shrimp-flavored instant noodles

- 3 teaspoons low sodium soy sauce

- ½ teaspoon ground ginger

Directions:

1. In a large skillet, melt the butter. Add the minced garlic, sweat it for 1 minute. Add the shrimp and vegetables to the skillet. Season with salt and pepper. Cover and simmer for 5 - 10 minutes, until the shrimp turns pink and the vegetables are tender.

2. Boil water in a separate pot. Add the noodles. Turn off the heat, cover the pot. Let it stand for 3 minutes. (Keep the water.)

3. Using a scoop or tongs, transfer the noodles to the skillet with the shrimp and vegetables. Stir in the seasoning packet. Mix, then serve immediately.

Nutrition:

Calories 80

Protein 18.9g

Carbohydrates 62g

Fat 9g

Sodium 276mg

Steamed Blue Crabs

Preparation time: 15 minutes

Cooking time: 10 minutes

Servings: 6

Ingredients:

- 30 live blue crabs

- ½ cup seafood seasoning

- ¼ cup of salt

- 3 cups beer

- 3 cups distilled white vinegar

Directions:

1. In a large stockpot, combine the seasoning, salt, beer, and white vinegar. Bring it to a boil. Put each crab upside down, then stick a knife into the shell just before cooking them. Cover the lid, leaving a crack for the steam to vent.

2. Steam the crabs until they turn bright orange and float to the top. Allow them to cook for another 2 - 3 minutes. Serve immediately.

Nutrition:

Calories 77

Protein 9.8g

Carbohydrates 31g

Fat 7g

Sodium 119mg

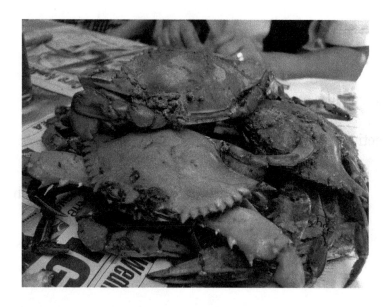

Ginger Sesame Salmon

Preparation time: 15 minutes

Cooking time: 5 minutes

Servings: 2

Ingredients:

- 4 ounces salmon

- ¼ cup low-sodium soy sauce

- 2 Tablespoons Balsamic vinegar

- ½ teaspoon sesame oil

- 2-inch chunk ginger, peeled and grated

- 1 garlic clove, minced

- 1 teaspoon flavorless oil (olive, canola, or sunflower)

- 1 teaspoon sesame seeds

- 1 teaspoon green onion, minced

Directions:

1. In a glass dish, combine the soy sauce, balsamic vinegar, sesame oil, garlic, and ginger. Place the salmon in the dish. Cover, marinate for 15 - 60 minutes in the fridge.

2. In a nonstick skillet, heat 1 teaspoon of oil. Sauté the fish until it becomes firm and golden on each side.

Sprinkle the sesame seeds in the pan. Heat for 1 minute. Serve immediately. Garnish with green onion.

Nutrition:

Calories 422

Protein 10.8g

Carbohydrates 5.7g

Fat 18g

Sodium 300mg

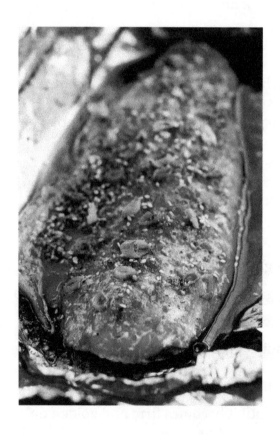

Sicilian Spaghetti with Tuna

Preparation time: 15 minutes

Cooking time: 10 minutes

Servings: 2

Ingredients:

- ½ cup fresh Tuna, cut into ½ inch pieces

- 85 grams whole wheat pasta

- ½ medium yellow onion, diced

- 1 garlic clove, minced

- ½ teaspoon anchovy paste

- ½ chipotle chili, minced

- 1 cup fresh tomatoes, chopped

- 1 teaspoon capers, drained and rinsed

- 1 cup fresh spinach, chopped

- ½ tablespoon fresh or dried marjoram

- 1 teaspoon flavorless oil (olive, canola, or sunflower)

Directions:

1. In a large skillet, drizzle oil over the bottom. Sweat the onion for 1 minute. Add the garlic, anchovy paste, and chipotle chili. Cook for 2 minutes.

2. Add the chopped tomatoes and capers. Sauté 2 minutes. Add the fresh spinach and tuna. Cover and cook for 2 - 5 minutes until the tuna is cooked. Turn off the heat. Sprinkle the mixture with the marjoram. Serve over cooked spaghetti.

Nutrition:

Calories 166

Protein 11g

Carbohydrates 112g

Fat 17.8g

Sodium 304mg

Poultry

Parmesan and Chicken Spaghetti Squash

Preparation time: 15 minutes

Cooking time: 20 minutes

Servings: 6

Ingredients:

- 16 oz. mozzarella

- 1 spaghetti squash piece

- 1 lb. cooked cube chicken

- 1 c. Marinara sauce

Directions:

1. Split up the squash in halves and remove the seeds. Arrange or put one cup of water in your pot, then put a trivet on top.

2. Add the squash halves to the trivet. Cook within 20 minutes at HIGH pressure. Remove the squashes and shred them using a fork into spaghetti portions

3. Pour sauce over the squash and give it a nice mix. Top them up with the cubed-up chicken and top

with mozzarella. Broil for 1-2 minutes and broil until the cheese has melted

Nutrition:

Calories: 237

Fat:10 g

Carbs:32 g

Protein:11 g

Sodium: 500 mg

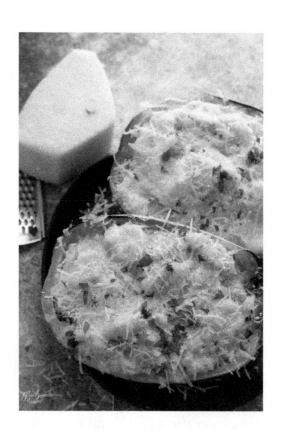

Apricot Chicken

Preparation time: 15 minutes

Cooking time: 6 minutes

Servings: 4

Ingredients:

- 1 bottle creamy French dressing

- ¼ c. flavorless oil

- White cooked rice

- 1 large jar Apricot preserve

- 4 lbs. boneless and skinless chicken

- 1 package onion soup mix

Directions:

1. Rinse and pat dry the chicken. Dice into bite-size pieces. In a large bowl, mix the apricot preserve, creamy dressing, and onion soup mix. Stir until thoroughly combined. Place the chicken in the bowl. Mix until coated.

2. In a large skillet, heat the oil. Place the chicken in the oil gently. Cook 4 – 6 minutes on each side, until golden brown. Serve over rice.

Nutrition:

Calories: 202

Fat:12 g

Carbs:75 g

Protein:20 g

Sugars:10 g

Sodium: 630 mg

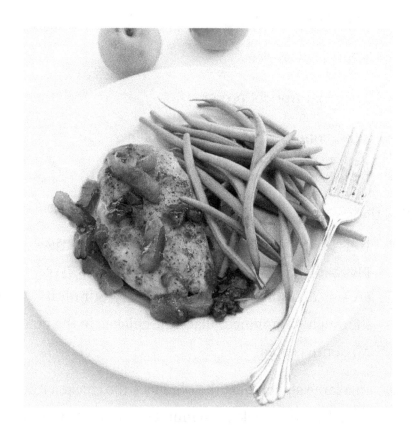

Oven-Fried Chicken Breasts

Preparation time: 15 minutes

Cooking time: 30 minutes

Servings: 8

Ingredients:

- ½ pack Ritz crackers

- 1 c. plain non-fat yogurt

- 8 boneless, skinless, and halved chicken breasts

Directions:

1. Preheat the oven to 350 0F. Rinse and pat dry the chicken breasts. Pour the yogurt into a shallow bowl. Dip the chicken pieces in the yogurt, then roll in the cracker crumbs. Place the chicken in a single layer in a baking dish. Bake within 15 minutes per side. Serve.

Nutrition:

Calories: 200

Fat:13 g

Carbs:98 g

Protein:19 g

Sodium:217 mg

Rosemary Roasted Chicken

Preparation time: 15 minutes

Cooking time: 20 minutes

Servings: 8

Ingredients:

- 8 rosemary springs

- 1 minced garlic clove

- Black pepper

- 1 tbsp. chopped rosemary

- 1 chicken

- 1 tbsp. organic olive oil

Directions:

1. In a bowl, mix garlic with rosemary, rub the chicken with black pepper, the oil and rosemary mix, place it inside roasting pan, introduce inside the oven at 350 0F, and roast for sixty minutes and 20 min. Carve chicken, divide between plates and serve using a side dish. Enjoy!

Nutrition:

Calories: 325

Fat:5 g

Carbs:15 g

Protein:14 g

Sodium: 950 mg

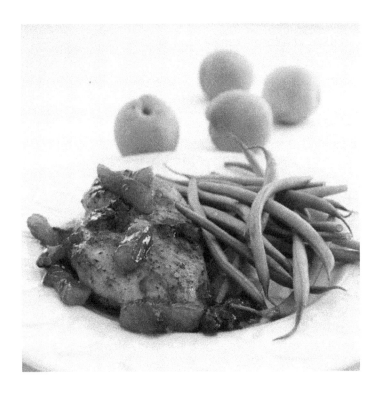

Artichoke and Spinach Chicken

Preparation time: 15 minutes

Cooking time: 5 minutes

Servings: 4

Ingredients:

- 10 oz baby spinach

- ½ tsp. crushed red pepper flakes

- 14 oz. chopped artichoke hearts

- 28 oz. no-salt-added tomato sauce

- 2 tbsps. Essential olive oil

- 4 boneless and skinless chicken breasts

Directions:

1. Heat-up a pan with the oil over medium-high heat, add chicken and red pepper flakes and cook for 5 minutes on them. Add spinach, artichokes, and tomato sauce, toss, cook for ten minutes more, divide between plates and serve. Enjoy!

Nutrition:

Calories: 212

Fat:3 g

Carbs:16 g

Protein:20 g

Sugars:5 g
Sodium:418 mg

Pumpkin and Black Beans Chicken

Preparation time: 15 minutes

Cooking time: 25 minutes

Servings: 4

Ingredients:

- 1 tbsp. essential olive oil

- 1 tbsp. Chopped cilantro

- 1 c. coconut milk

- 15 oz canned black beans, drained

- 1 lb. skinless and boneless chicken breasts

- 2 c. water

- ½ c. pumpkin flesh

Directions:

1. Heat a pan when using oil over medium-high heat, add the chicken and cook for 5 minutes. Add the river, milk, pumpkin, and black beans toss, cover the pan, reduce heat to medium and cook for 20 mins. Add cilantro, toss, divide between plates and serve. Enjoy!

Nutrition:

Calories: 254

Fat:6 g

Carbs:16 g

Protein:22 g

Sodium:92 mg

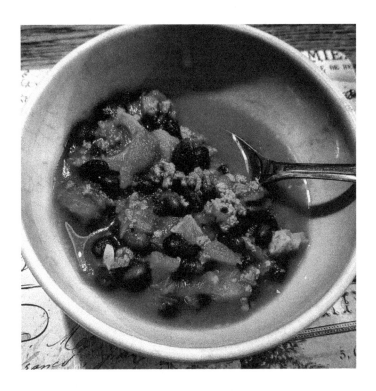

Chicken Thighs and Apples Mix

Preparation time: 15 minutes

Cooking time: 60 minutes

Servings: 4

Ingredients:

- 3 cored and sliced apples

- 1 tbsp apple cider vinegar treatment

- ¾ c. natural apple juice

- ¼ tsp. pepper and salt

- 1 tbsp. grated ginger

- 8 chicken thighs

- 3 tbsps. Chopped onion

Directions:

1. In a bowl, mix chicken with salt, pepper, vinegar, onion, ginger, and apple juice, toss well, cover, keep within the fridge for ten minutes, transfer with a baking dish, and include apples. Introduce inside the oven at 400 0F for just 1 hour. Divide between plates and serve. Enjoy!

Nutrition:

Calories: 214

Fat:3 g

Carbs:14 g

Protein:15 g

Sodium:405 mg

Thai Chicken Thighs

Preparation time: 15 minutes

Cooking time: 1 hour & 5minutes

Servings: 6

Ingredients:

- ½ c. Thai chili sauce

- 1 chopped green onions bunch

- 4 lbs. chicken thighs

Directions:

1. Heat a pan over medium-high heat. Add chicken thighs, brown them for 5 minutes on both sides Transfer to some baking dish, then add chili sauce and green onions and toss.

2. Introduce within the oven and bake at 4000F for 60 minutes. Divide everything between plates and serve. Enjoy!

Nutrition:

Calories: 220

Fat:4 g

Carbs:12 g

Protein:10 g

Sodium: 870 mg

Falling "Off" The Bone Chicken

Preparation time: 15 minutes

Cooking time: 40 minutes

Servings: 4

Ingredients:

- 6 peeled garlic cloves

- 1 tbsp. organic extra virgin coconut oil

- 2 tbsps. Lemon juice

- 1 ½ c. pacific organic bone chicken broth

- ¼ tsp freshly ground black pepper

- ½ tsp. sea flavored vinegar

- 1 whole organic chicken piece

- 1 tsp. paprika

- 1 tsp. dried thyme

Directions:

1. Take a small bowl and toss in the thyme, paprika, pepper, and flavored vinegar and mix them. Use the mixture to season the chicken properly. Pour down the oil in your instant pot and heat it to shimmering; toss in the chicken with breast downward and let it cook for about 6-7 minutes

2. After the 7 minutes, flip over the chicken pour down the broth, garlic cloves, and lemon juice. Cook within 25 minutes on a high setting. Remove the dish from the cooker and let it stand for about 5 minutes before serving.

Nutrition:

Calories: 664

Fat:44 g

Carbs:44 g

Protein:27 g

Sugars:0.1 g

Sodium:800 mg

Feisty Chicken Porridge

Preparation time: 15 minutes

Cooking time: 30 minutes

Servings: 4

Ingredients:

- 1 ½ c. fresh ginger

- 1 lb. cooked chicken legs

- Green onions

- Toasted cashew nuts

- 5 c. chicken broth

- 1 cup jasmine rice

- 4 c. water

Directions:

1. Place the rice in your fridge and allow it to chill 1 hour before cooking. Take the rice out and add them to your Instant Pot. Pour broth and water. Lock up the lid and cook on Porridge mode.

2. Separate the meat from the chicken legs and add the meat to your soup. Stir well over sauté mode. Season with a bit of flavored vinegar and enjoy with a garnish of nuts and onion

Nutrition:

Calories: 206

Fat:8 g

Carbs:8 g

Protein:23 g

Sugars:0 g

Sodium:950 mg

The Ultimate Faux-Tisserie Chicken

Preparation time: 15 minutes

Cooking time: 35 minutes

Servings: 5

Ingredients:

- 1 c. low sodium broth

- 2 tbsps. Olive oil

- ½ quartered medium onion

- 2 tbsps. Favorite seasoning

- 2 ½ lbs. whole chicken

- Black pepper

- 5 large fresh garlic cloves

Directions:

1. Massage the chicken with 1 tablespoon of olive oil and sprinkle pepper on top. Place onion wedges and garlic cloves inside the chicken. Take a butcher's twin and secure the legs

2. Set your pot to Sauté mode. Put olive oil in your pan on medium heat, allow the oil to heat up. Add chicken and sear both sides for 4 minutes per side. Sprinkle your seasoning over the chicken, remove

the chicken and place a trivet at the bottom of your pot

3. Sprinkle seasoning over the chicken, making sure to rub it. Transfer the chicken to the trivet with the breast side facing up, lock up the lid. Cook on HIGH pressure for 25 minutes. Allow it to rest and serve!

Nutrition:

Calories: 1010

Fat:64 g

Carbs:47 g

Protein:60 g

Sodium:209 mg

Oregano Chicken Thighs

Preparation time: 15 minutes

Cooking time: 20 minutes

Servings: 6

Ingredients:

- 12 chicken thighs

- 1 tsp dried parsley

- ¼ tsp. pepper and salt.

- ½ c. extra virgin essential olive oil

- 4 minced garlic cloves

- 1 c. chopped oregano

- ¼ c. low-sodium veggie stock

Directions:

1. In your food processor, mix parsley with oregano, garlic, salt, pepper, and stock and pulse. Put chicken thighs within the bowl, add oregano paste, toss, cover, and then leave aside within the fridge for 10 minutes.

2. Heat the kitchen grill over medium heat, add chicken pieces, close the lid and cook for twenty or so minutes with them. Divide between plates and serve!

Nutrition:

Calories: 254

Fat:3 g

Carbs:7 g

Protein:17 g

Sugars:0.9 g

Sodium:730 mg

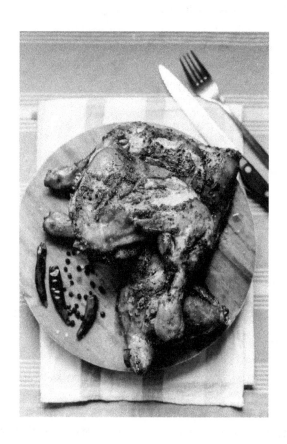

Pesto Chicken Breasts with Summer Squash

Preparation time: 15 minutes

Cooking time: 10 minutes

Servings: 4

Ingredients:

- 4 medium boneless, skinless chicken breast halves

- 1 tbsp. olive oil

- 2 tbsps. Homemade pesto

- 2 c. finely chopped zucchini

- 2 tbsps. Finely shredded Asiago

Directions:

1. Cook your chicken in hot oil on medium heat within 4 minutes in a large nonstick skillet. Flip the chicken then put the zucchini.

2. Cook within 4 to 6 minutes more or until the chicken is tender and no longer pink (170 F), and squash is crisp-tender, stirring squash gently once or twice. Transfer chicken and squash to 4 dinner plates. Spread pesto over chicken; sprinkle with Asiago.

Nutrition:

Calories: 230
Fat:9 g
Carbs:8 g
Protein:30 g
Sodium:578 mg

Chicken, Tomato and Green Beans

Preparation time: 15 minutes

Cooking time: 25 minutes

Servings: 4

Ingredients:

- 6 oz. low-sodium canned tomato paste

- 2 tbsps. Olive oil

- ¼ tsp. black pepper

- 2 lbs. trimmed green beans

- 2 tbsps. Chopped parsley

- 1 ½ lbs. boneless, skinless, and cubed chicken breasts

- 25 oz. no-salt-added canned tomato sauce

Directions:

1. Heat a pan with 50 % with the oil over medium heat, add chicken, stir, cover, cook within 5 minutes on both sides and transfer to a bowl. Heat inside the same pan while using rest through the oil over medium heat, add green beans, stir and cook for 10 minutes.

2. Return chicken for that pan, add black pepper, tomato sauce, tomato paste, and parsley, stir, cover,

cook for 10 minutes more, divide between plates and serve. Enjoy!

Nutrition:

Calories: 190

Fat:4 g

Carbs:12 g

Protein:9 g

Sodium:168 mg

Chicken Tortillas

Preparation time: 15 minutes

Cooking time: 5 minutes

Servings: 4

Ingredients:

- 6 oz. boneless, skinless, and cooked chicken breasts

- Black pepper

- 1/3 c. fat-free yogurt

- 4 heated up whole-wheat tortillas

- 2 chopped tomatoes

Directions:

1. Heat-up a pan over medium heat, add one tortilla during those times, heat up, and hang them on the working surface. Spread yogurt on each tortilla, add chicken and tomatoes, roll, divide between plates and serve. Enjoy!

Nutrition:

Calories:190

Fat:2 g

Carbs:12 g

Protein:6 g

Sodium:300 mg

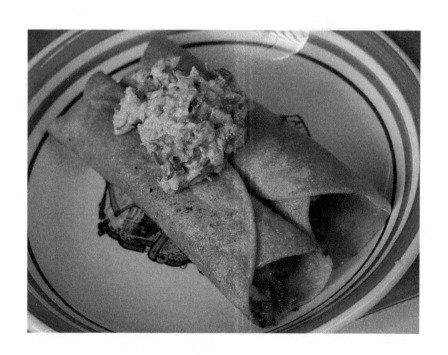

Chicken with Potatoes Olives & Sprouts

Preparation time: 15 minutes

Cooking time: 35 minutes

Servings: 4

Ingredients:

- 1 lb. chicken breasts, skinless, boneless, and cut into pieces

- ¼ cup olives, quartered

- 1 tsp oregano

- 1 ½ tsp Dijon mustard

- 1 lemon juice

- 1/3 cup vinaigrette dressing

- 1 medium onion, diced

- 3 cups potatoes cut into pieces

- 4 cups Brussels sprouts, trimmed and quartered

- ¼ tsp pepper

- ¼ tsp salt

Directions:

1. Warm-up oven to 400 F. Place chicken in the center of the baking tray, then place potatoes, sprouts, and onions around the chicken.

2. In a small bowl, mix vinaigrette, oregano, mustard, lemon juice, and salt and pour over chicken and veggies. Sprinkle olives and season with pepper.

3. Bake in preheated oven for 20 minutes. Transfer chicken to a plate. Stir the vegetables and roast for 15 minutes more. Serve and enjoy.

Nutrition:

Calories: 397

Fat: 13g

Protein: 38.3g

Carbs: 31.4g

Sodium 175 mg

Garlic Mushroom Chicken

Preparation time: 15 minutes

Cooking time: 15 minutes

Servings: 4

Ingredients:

- 4 chicken breasts, boneless and skinless

- 3 garlic cloves, minced

- 1 onion, chopped

- 2 cups mushrooms, sliced

- 1 tbsp olive oil

- ½ cup chicken stock

- ¼ tsp pepper

- ½ tsp salt

Directions:

1. Season chicken with pepper and salt. Warm oil in a pan on medium heat, then put season chicken in the pan and cook for 5-6 minutes on each side. Remove and place on a plate.

2. Add onion and mushrooms to the pan and sauté until tender, about 2-3 minutes. Add garlic and sauté for a minute. Add stock and bring to boil. Stir

well and cook for 1-2 minutes. Pour over chicken and serve.

Nutrition:

Calories: 331

Fat: 14.5g

Protein: 43.9g

Carbs: 4.6g

Sodium 420 mg

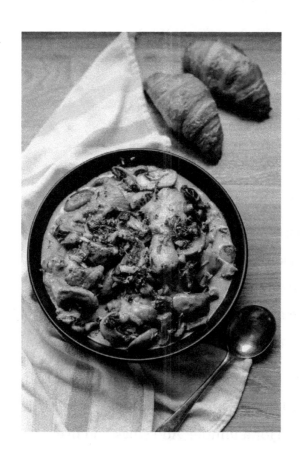

Grilled Chicken

Preparation time: 15 minutes

Cooking time: 15 minutes

Servings: 4

Ingredients:

- 4 chicken breasts, skinless and boneless
- 1 ½ tsp dried oregano
- 1 tsp paprika
- 5 garlic cloves, minced
- ½ cup fresh parsley, minced
- ½ cup olive oil
- ½ cup fresh lemon juice
- Pepper
- Salt

Directions:

1. Add lemon juice, oregano, paprika, garlic, parsley, and olive oil to a large zip-lock bag. Season chicken with pepper and salt and add to bag. Seal bag and shake well to coat chicken with marinade. Let sit chicken in the marinade for 20 minutes.

2. Remove chicken from marinade and grill over medium-high heat for 5-6 minutes on each side. Serve and enjoy.

Nutrition:

Calories: 512

Fat: 36.5g

Protein: 43.1g

Carbs: 3g

Sodium 110mg

Delicious Lemon Chicken Salad

Preparation time: 15 minutes

Cooking time: 5 minutes

Servings: 4

Ingredients:

- 1 lb. chicken breast, cooked and diced

- 1 tbsp fresh dill, chopped

- 2 tsp olive oil

- 1/4 cup low-fat yogurt

- 1 tsp lemon zest, grated

- 2 tbsp onion, minced

- ¼ tsp pepper

- ¼ tsp salt

Directions:

1. Put all your fixing into the large mixing bowl and toss well. Season with pepper and salt. Cover and place in the refrigerator. Serve chilled and enjoy.

Nutrition:

Calories: 165

Fat: 5.4g

Protein: 25.2g

Carbs: 2.2g

Sodium 153mg

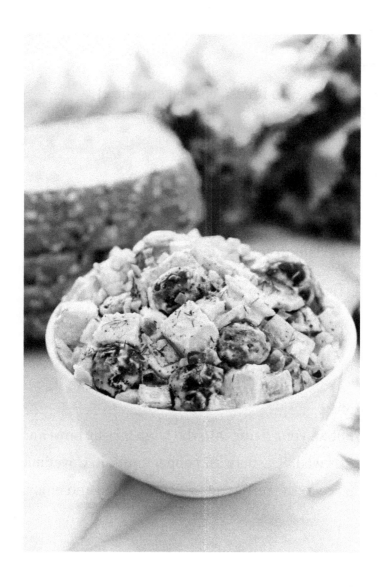

Healthy Chicken Orzo

Preparation time: 15 minutes

Cooking time: 15 minutes

Servings: 4

Ingredients:

- 1 cup whole wheat orzo

- 1 lb. chicken breasts, sliced

- ½ tsp red pepper flakes

- ½ cup feta cheese, crumbled

- ½ tsp oregano

- 1 tbsp fresh parsley, chopped

- 1 tbsp fresh basil, chopped

- ¼ cup pine nuts

- 1 cup spinach, chopped

- ¼ cup white wine

- ½ cup olives, sliced

- 1 cup grape tomatoes, cut in half

- ½ tbsp garlic, minced

- 2 tbsp olive oil

- ½ tsp pepper

- ½ tsp salt

Directions:

1. Add water in a small saucepan and bring to boil. Heat 1 tablespoon of olive oil in a pan over medium heat. Season chicken with pepper and salt and cook in the pan for 5-7 minutes on each side. Remove from pan and set aside.

2. Add orzo in boiling water and cook according to the packet directions. Heat remaining olive oil in a pan on medium heat, then put garlic in the pan and sauté for a minute. Stir in white wine and cherry tomatoes and cook on high for 3 minutes.

3. Add cooked orzo, spices, spinach, pine nuts, and olives and stir until well combined. Add chicken on top of orzo and sprinkle with feta cheese. Serve and enjoy.

Nutrition:

Calories: 518

Fat: 27.7g

Protein: 40.6g

Carbs: 26.2g

Sodium 121mg

Lemon Garlic Chicken

Preparation time: 15 minutes

Cooking time: 12 minutes

Servings: 3

Ingredients:

- 3 chicken breasts, cut into thin slices

- 2 lemon zest, grated

- ¼ cup olive oil

- 4 garlic cloves, minced

- Pepper

- Salt

Directions:

1. Warm-up olive oil in a pan over medium heat. Add garlic to the pan and sauté for 30 seconds. Put the chicken in the pan and sauté within 10 minutes. Add lemon zest and lemon juice and bring to boil. Remove from heat and season with pepper and salt. Serve and enjoy.

Nutrition:

Calories: 439

Fat: 27.8g

Protein: 42.9g

Carbs: 4.9g

Sodium 306 mg

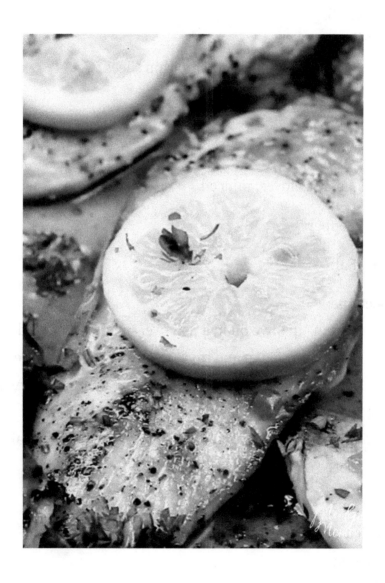

Simple Mediterranean Chicken

Preparation time: 15 minutes

Cooking time: 15 minutes

Servings: 12

Ingredients:

- 2 chicken breasts, skinless and boneless

- 1 ½ cup grape tomatoes, cut in half

- ½ cup olives

- 2 tbsp olive oil

- 1 tsp Italian seasoning

- ¼ tsp pepper

- ¼ tsp salt

Directions:

1. Season chicken with Italian seasoning, pepper, and salt. Warm-up olive oil in a pan over medium heat. Add season chicken to the pan and cook for 4-6 minutes on each side. Transfer chicken on a plate.

2. Put tomatoes plus olives in the pan and cook for 2-4 minutes. Pour olive and tomato mixture on top of the chicken and serve.

Nutrition:

Calories: 468

Fat: 29.4g

Protein: 43.8g

Carbs: 7.8g

Sodium 410 mg

Roasted Chicken Thighs

Preparation time: 15 minutes

Cooking time: 55 minutes

Servings: 4

Ingredients:

- 8 chicken thighs

- 3 tbsp fresh parsley, chopped

- 1 tsp dried oregano

- 6 garlic cloves, crushed

- ¼ cup capers, drained

- 10 oz roasted red peppers, sliced

- 2 cups grape tomatoes

- 1 ½ lbs. potatoes, cut into small chunks

- 4 tbsp olive oil

- Pepper

- Salt

Directions:

1. Warm oven to 200 400 F. Season chicken with pepper and salt. Heat-up 2 tablespoons of olive oil in a pan over medium heat. Add chicken to the pan and sear until lightly golden brown from all the sides.

2. Transfer chicken onto a baking tray. Add tomato,
    potatoes, capers, oregano, garlic, and red peppers
    around the chicken. Season with pepper and salt and
    drizzle with remaining olive oil. Bake in preheated
    oven for 45-55 minutes. Garnish with parsley and
    serve.

Nutrition:

Calories: 848

Fat: 29.1g

Protein: 91.3g

Carbs: 45.2g

Sodium 110 mg

Mediterranean Turkey Breast

Preparation time: 15 minutes

Cooking time: 4 minutes & 30 minutes

Servings: 6

Ingredients:

- 4 lbs. turkey breast

- 3 tbsp flour

- ¾ cup chicken stock

- 4 garlic cloves, chopped

- 1 tsp dried oregano

- ½ fresh lemon juice

- ½ cup sun-dried tomatoes, chopped

- ½ cup olives, chopped

- 1 onion, chopped

- ¼ tsp pepper

- ½ tsp salt

Directions:

1. Add turkey breast, garlic, oregano, lemon juice, sun-dried tomatoes, olives, onion, pepper, and salt to the slow cooker. Add half stock. Cook on high within 4 hours.

2. Whisk remaining stock and flour in a small bowl and add to slow cooker. Cover and cook for 30 minutes more. Serve and enjoy.

Nutrition:

Calories: 537

Fat: 9.7g

Protein: 79.1g

Carbs: 29.6g

Sodium 330 mg

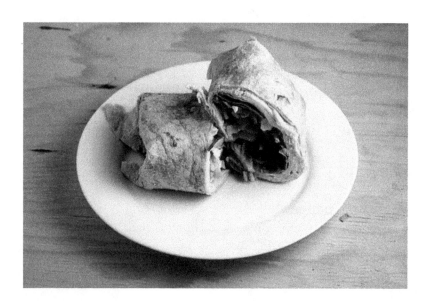

Olive Capers Chicken

Preparation time: 15 minutes

Cooking time: 16 minutes

Servings: 4

Ingredients:

- 2 lbs. chicken

- 1/3 cup chicken stock

- 3.5 oz Capers

- 6 oz olives

- 1/4 cup fresh basil

- 1 tbsp olive oil

- 1 tsp oregano

- 2 garlic cloves, minced

- 2 tbsp red wine vinegar

- 1/8 tsp pepper

- 1/4 tsp salt

Directions:

1. Put olive oil in your instant pot and set the pot on sauté mode. Add chicken to the pot and sauté for 3-4 minutes. Add remaining ingredients and stir well.

Seal pot with the lid and select manual, and set timer for 12 minutes. Serve and enjoy.

Nutrition:

Calories: 433

Fat: 15.2g

Protein: 66.9g

Carbs: 4.8g

Sodium 244 mg

Chicken with Mushrooms

Preparation time: 15 minutes

Cooking time: 6 hours & 10 minutes

Servings: 2

Ingredients:

- 2 chicken breasts, skinless and boneless

- 1 cup mushrooms, sliced

- 1 onion, sliced

- 1 cup chicken stock

- 1/2 tsp thyme, dried

- Pepper

- Salt

Directions:

1. Add all ingredients to the slow cooker. Cook on low within 6 hours. Serve and enjoy.

Nutrition:

Calories: 313

Fat: 11.3g

Protein: 44.3g

Carbs: 6.9g

Sodium 541 mg

Baked Chicken

Preparation time: 15 minutes

Cooking time: 35 minutes

Servings: 4

Ingredients:

- 2 lbs. chicken tenders

- 1 large zucchini

- 1 cup grape tomatoes

- 2 tbsp olive oil

- 3 dill sprigs

For topping:

- 2 tbsp feta cheese, crumbled

- 1 tbsp olive oil

- 1 tbsp fresh lemon juice

- 1 tbsp fresh dill, chopped

Directions:

1. Warm oven to 200 C/ 400 F. Drizzle the olive oil on a baking tray, then place chicken, zucchini, dill, and tomatoes on the tray. Season with salt. Bake chicken within 30 minutes.

2. Meanwhile, in a small bowl, stir all topping ingredients. Place chicken on the serving tray, then top with veggies and discard dill sprigs. Sprinkle topping mixture on top of chicken and vegetables. Serve and enjoy.

Nutrition:

Calories: 557

Fat: 28.6g

Protein: 67.9g

Carbs: 5.2g

Sodium 760 mg

Garlic Pepper Chicken

Preparation time: 15 minutes

Cooking time: 21 minutes

Servings: 2

Ingredients:

- 2 chicken breasts, cut into strips

- 2 bell peppers, cut into strips

- 5 garlic cloves, chopped

- 3 tbsp water

- 2 tbsp olive oil

- 1 tbsp paprika

- 2 tsp black pepper

- 1/2 tsp salt

Directions:

1. Warm-up olive oil in a large saucepan over medium heat. Add garlic and sauté for 2-3 minutes. Add peppers and cook for 3 minutes. Add chicken and spices and stir to coat. Add water and stir well. Bring to boil. Cover and simmer for 10-15 minutes. Serve and enjoy.

Nutrition:

Calories: 462

Fat: 25.7g

Protein: 44.7g

Carbs: 14.8g

Sodium 720 mg

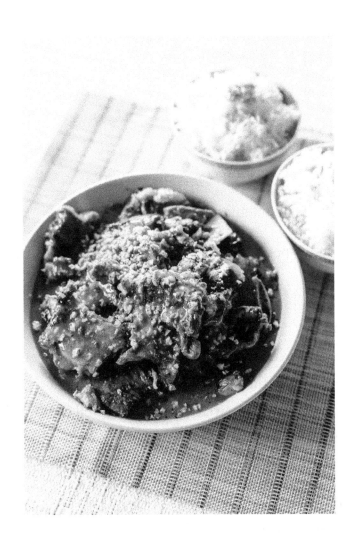

Mustard Chicken Tenders

Preparation time: 15 minutes

Cooking time: 20 minutes

Servings: 4

Ingredients:

- 1 lb. chicken tenders

- 2 tbsp fresh tarragon, chopped

- 1/2 cup whole grain mustard

- 1/2 tsp paprika

- 1 garlic clove, minced

- 1/2 oz fresh lemon juice

- 1/2 tsp pepper

- 1/4 tsp kosher salt

Directions:

1. Warm oven to 425 F. Add all ingredients except chicken to the large bowl and mix well. Put the chicken in the bowl, then stir until well coated. Place chicken on a baking dish and cover. Bake within 15-20 minutes. Serve and enjoy.

Nutrition:

Calories: 242

Fat: 9.5g

Protein: 33.2g

Carbs: 3.1g

Sodium 240 mg

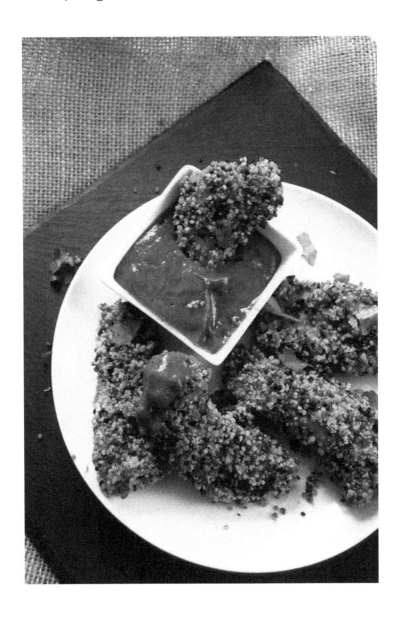

Salsa Chicken Chili

Preparation time: 15 minutes

Cooking time: 20 minutes

Servings: 8

Ingredients:

- 2 1/2 lbs. chicken breasts, skinless and boneless

- 1/2 tsp cumin powder

- 3 garlic cloves, minced

- 1 onion, diced

- 16 oz salsa

- 1 tsp oregano

- 1 tbsp olive oil

Directions:

1. Add oil into the instant pot and set the pot on sauté mode. Add onion to the pot and sauté until softened, about 3 minutes. Add garlic and sauté for a minute. Add oregano and cumin and sauté for a minute. Add half salsa and stir well. Place chicken and pour remaining salsa over chicken.

2. Seal pot with the lid and select manual, and set timer for 10 minutes. Remove chicken and shred.

Move it back to the pot, then stir well to combine.
Serve and enjoy.

Nutrition:

Calories: 308

Fat: 12.4g

Protein: 42.1g

Carbs: 5.4g

Sodium 656 mg

Honey Crusted Chicken

Preparation time: 10 minutes

Cooking time: 25 minutes

Servings: 2

Ingredients:

- 1 teaspoon paprika

- 8 saltine crackers, 2 inches square

- 2 chicken breasts, each 4 ounces

- 4 tsp honey

Directions:

1. Set the oven to heat at 375 degrees F. Grease a baking dish with cooking oil. Smash the crackers in a Ziplock bag and toss them with paprika in a bowl. Brush chicken with honey and add it to the crackers.

2. Mix well and transfer the chicken to the baking dish. Bake the chicken for 25 minutes until golden brown. Serve.

Nutrition:

Calories 219

Fat 17 g

Sodium 456 mg

Carbs 12.1 g

Protein 31 g

Paella with Chicken, Leeks, and Tarragon

Preparation time: 10 minutes

Cooking time: 20 minutes

Servings: 2

Ingredients:

- 1 teaspoon extra-virgin olive oil

- 1 small onion, sliced

- 2 leeks (whites only), thinly sliced

- 3 garlic cloves, minced

- 1-pound boneless, skinless chicken breast, cut into strips 1/2-inch-wide and 2 inches long

- 2 large tomatoes, chopped

- 1 red pepper, sliced

- 2/3 cup long-grain brown rice

- 1 teaspoon tarragon, or to taste

- 2 cups fat-free, unsalted chicken broth

- 1 cup frozen peas

- 1/4 cup chopped fresh parsley

- 1 lemon, cut into 4 wedges

Directions:

1. Preheat a nonstick pan with olive oil over medium heat. Toss in leeks, onions, chicken strips, and garlic. Sauté for 5 minutes. Stir in red pepper slices and tomatoes. Stir and cook for 5 minutes.

2. Add tarragon, broth, and rice. Let it boil, then reduce the heat to a simmer. Continue cooking for 10 minutes, then add peas and continue cooking until the liquid is thoroughly cooked. Garnish with parsley and lemon. Serve.

Nutrition:

Calories 388

Fat 15.2 g

Sodium 572 mg

Carbs 5.4 g

Protein 27 g

Southwestern Chicken and Pasta

Preparation time: 10 minutes

Cooking time: 10 minutes

Servings: 2

Ingredients:

- 1 cup uncooked whole-wheat rigatoni

- 2 chicken breasts, cut into cubes

- 1/4 cup of salsa

- 1 1/2 cups of canned unsalted tomato sauce

- 1/8 tsp garlic powder

- 1 tsp cumin

- 1/2 tsp chili powder

- 1/2 cup canned black beans, drained

- 1/2 cup fresh corn

- 1/4 cup Monterey Jack and Colby cheese, shredded

Directions:

1. Fill a pot with water up to ¾ full and boil it. Add pasta to cook until it is al dente, then drain the pasta while rinsing under cold water. Preheat a skillet with cooking oil, then cook the chicken for 10 minutes until golden from both sides.

2. Add tomato sauce, salsa, cumin, garlic powder, black beans, corn, and chili powder. Cook the mixture while stirring, then toss in the pasta. Serve with 2 tablespoons cheese on top. Enjoy.

Nutrition:

Calories 245

Fat 16.3 g

Sodium 515 mg

Carbs 19.3 g

Protein 33.3 g

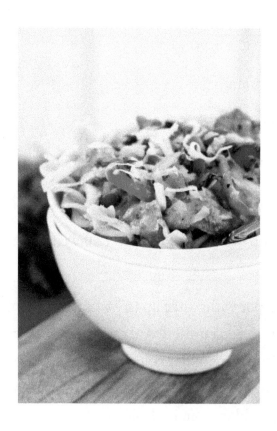

Stuffed Chicken Breasts

Preparation time: 15 minutes

Cooking time: 30 minutes

Servings: 4

Ingredients:

- 3 tbsp seedless raisins

- 1/2 cup of chopped onion

- 1/2 cup of chopped celery

- 1/4 tsp garlic, minced

- 1 bay leaf

- 1 cup apple with peel, chopped

- 2 tbsp chopped water chestnuts

- 4 large chicken breast halves, 5 ounces each

- 1 tablespoon olive oil

- 1 cup fat-free milk

- 1 teaspoon curry powder

- 2 tablespoons all-purpose (plain) flour

- 1 lemon, cut into 4 wedges

Directions:

1. Set the oven to heat at 425 degrees F. Grease a baking dish with cooking oil. Soak raisins in warm water until they swell. Grease a heated skillet with cooking spray.

2. Add celery, garlic, onions, and bay leaf. Sauté for 5 minutes. Discard the bay leaf, then toss in apples. Stir cook for 2 minutes. Drain the soaked raisin and pat them dry to remove excess water.

3. Add raisins and water chestnuts to the apple mixture. Pull apart the chicken's skin and stuff the apple raisin mixture between the skin and the chicken. Preheat olive oil in another skillet and sear the breasts for 5 minutes per side.

4. Place the chicken breasts in the baking dish and cover the dish. Bake for 15 minutes until temperature reaches 165 degrees F. Prepare sauce by mixing milk, flour, and curry powder in a saucepan.

5. Stir cook until the mixture thickens, about 5 minutes. Pour this sauce over the baked chicken. Bake again in the covered dish for 10 minutes. Serve.

Nutrition:

Calories 357

Fat 32.7 g

Sodium 277 mg

Carbs 17.7 g

Protein 31.2 g

Buffalo Chicken Salad Wrap

Preparation time: 10 minutes

Cooking time: 10 minutes

Servings: 4

Ingredients:

- 3-4 ounces chicken breasts

- 2 whole chipotle peppers

- 1/4 cup white wine vinegar

- 1/4 cup low-calorie mayonnaise

- 2 stalks celery, diced

- 2 carrots, cut into matchsticks

- 1 small yellow onion, diced

- 1/2 cup thinly sliced rutabaga or another root vegetable

- 4 ounces spinach, cut into strips

- 2 whole-grain tortillas (12-inch diameter)

Directions:

1. Set the oven or a grill to heat at 375 degrees F. Bake the chicken first for 10 minutes per side. Blend chipotle peppers with mayonnaise and wine vinegar

in the blender. Dice the baked chicken into cubes or small chunks.

2. Mix the chipotle mixture with all the ingredients except tortillas and spinach. Spread 2 ounces of spinach over the tortilla and scoop the stuffing on top. Wrap the tortilla and cut it into half. Serve.

Nutrition:

Calories 300

Fat 16.4 g

Sodium 471 mg

Carbs 8.7 g

Protein 38.5 g

Chicken Sliders

Preparation time: 10 minutes

Cooking time: 10 minutes

Servings: 4

Ingredients:

- 10 ounces ground chicken breast

- 1 tablespoon black pepper

- 1 tablespoon minced garlic

- 1 tablespoon balsamic vinegar

- 1/2 cup minced onion

- 1 fresh chili pepper, minced

- 1 tablespoon fennel seed, crushed

- 4 whole-wheat mini buns

- 4 lettuce leaves

- 4 tomato slices

Directions:

1. Combine all the ingredients except the wheat buns, tomato, and lettuce. Mix well and refrigerate the mixture for 1 hour. Divide the mixture into 4 patties.

2. Broil these patties in a greased baking tray until golden brown. Place the chicken patties in the wheat buns along with lettuce and tomato. Serve.

Nutrition:

Calories 224

Fat 4.5 g

Sodium 212 mg

Carbs 10.2 g

Protein 67.4 g

White Chicken Chili

Preparation time: 20 minutes

Cooking time: 15 minutes

Servings: 4

Ingredients:

- 1 can white chunk chicken

- 2 cans low-sodium white beans, drained

- 1 can low-sodium diced tomatoes

- 4 cups of low-sodium chicken broth

- 1 medium onion, chopped

- 1/2 medium green pepper, chopped

- 1 medium red pepper, chopped

- 2 garlic cloves, minced

- 2 teaspoons chili powder

- 1 teaspoon ground cumin

- 1 teaspoon dried oregano

- Cayenne pepper, to taste

- 8 tablespoons shredded reduced-fat Monterey Jack cheese

- 3 tablespoons chopped fresh cilantro

Directions:

1. In a soup pot, add beans, tomatoes, chicken, and chicken broth. Cover this soup pot and let it simmer over medium heat. Meanwhile, grease a nonstick pan with cooking spray. Add peppers, garlic, and onions. Sauté for 5 minutes until soft.

2. Transfer the mixture to the soup pot. Add cumin, chili powder, cayenne pepper, and oregano. Cook for 10 minutes, then garnish the chili with cilantro and 1 tablespoon cheese. Serve.

Nutrition:

Calories 225

Fat 12.9 g

Sodium 480 mg

Carbs 24.7 g

Protein 25.3g

Sweet Potato-Turkey Meatloaf

Preparation time: 15 minutes

Cooking time: 25 minutes

Servings: 4

Ingredients:

- 1 large sweet potato, peeled and cubed

- 1-pound ground turkey (breast)

- 1 large egg

- 1 small sweet onion, finely chopped

- 2 cloves garlic, minced

- 2 slices whole-wheat bread, crumbs

- ¼ cup honey barbecue sauce

- ¼ cup ketchup

- 2 Tablespoons Dijon Mustard

- 1 Tablespoon fresh ground pepper

- ½ Tablespoon salt

Directions:

1. Warm oven to 350 F. Grease a baking dish. In a large pot, boil a cup of lightly salted water, add the sweet potato. Cook until tender. Drain the water. Mash the potato.

2. Mix the honey barbecue sauce, ketchup, and Dijon mustard in a small bowl. Mix thoroughly. In a large bowl, mix the turkey and the egg. Add the sweet onion, garlic. Pour in the combined sauces. Add the bread crumbs. Season the mixture with salt and pepper.

3. Add the sweet potato. Combine thoroughly with your hands. If the mixture feels wet, add more bread crumbs. Shape the mixture into a loaf. Place in the loaf pan. Bake for 25 – 35 minutes until the meat is cooked through. Broil for 5 minutes. Slice and serve.

Nutrition:

Calories - 133

Protein - 85g

Carbohydrates - 50g

Fat - 34g

Sodium - 202mg

Oaxacan Chicken

Preparation time: 15 minutes

Cooking time: 28 minutes

Servings: 2

Ingredients:

- 1 4-ounce chicken breast, skinned and halved

- ½ cup uncooked long-grain rice

- 1 teaspoon of extra-virgin olive oil

- ½ cup low-sodium salsa

- ½ cup chicken stock, mixed with 2 Tablespoons water

- ¾ cup baby carrots

- 2 tablespoons green olives, pitted and chopped

- 2 Tablespoons dark raisins

- ½ teaspoon ground Cinnamon

- 2 Tablespoons fresh cilantro or parsley, coarsely chopped

Directions:

1. Warm oven to 350 F. In a large saucepan that can go in the oven, heat the olive oil. Add the rice. Sauté the rice until it begins to pop, approximately 2 minutes.

2. Add the salsa, baby carrots, green olives, dark raisins, halved chicken breast, chicken stock, and ground cinnamon. Bring the mix to a simmer, stir once.

3. Cover the mixture tightly, bake in the oven until the chicken stock has been completely absorbed, approximately 25 minutes. Sprinkle fresh cilantro or parsley, mix. Serve immediately.

Nutrition:

Calories - 143

Protein - 102g

Carbohydrates - 66g

Fat - 18g

Sodium - 97mg

Spicy Chicken with Minty Couscous

Preparation time: 15 minutes

Cooking time: 25 minutes

Servings: 2

Ingredients:

- 2 small chicken breasts, sliced

- 1 red chili pepper, finely chopped

- 1 garlic clove, crushed

- ginger root, 2 cm long peeled and grated

- 1 teaspoon ground cumin

- ½ teaspoon turmeric

- 2 Tablespoons extra-virgin olive oil

- 1 pinch sea salt

- ¾ cup couscous

- Small bunch mint leaves, finely chopped

- 2 lemons, grate the rind and juice them

Directions:

1. In a large bowl, place the chicken breast slices and chopped chili pepper. Sprinkle with the crushed garlic, ginger, cumin, turmeric, and a pinch of salt. Add the grated rind of both lemons and the juice

from 1 lemon. Pour 1 tablespoon of the olive oil over the chicken, coat evenly.

2. Cover the dish with plastic and refrigerate within 1 hour. After 1 hour, coat a skillet with olive oil and fry the chicken. As the chicken is cooking, pour the couscous into a bowl and pour hot water over it, let it absorb the water (approximately 5 minutes).

3. Fluff the couscous. Add some chopped mint, the other tablespoon of olive oil, and juice from the second lemon. Top the couscous with the chicken. Garnish with chopped mint. Serve immediately.

Nutrition:

Calories - 166

Protein - 106g

Carbohydrates - 52g

Sugars - 0.1g

Fat - 17g

Sodium - 108mg

Chicken, Pasta and Snow Peas

Preparation time: 15 minutes

Cooking time: 20 minutes

Servings: 2

Ingredients:

- 1-pound chicken breasts

- 2 ½ cups penne pasta

- 1 cup snow peas, trimmed and halved

- 1 teaspoon olive oil

- 1 standard jar Tomato and Basil pasta sauce

- Fresh ground pepper

Directions:

1. In a medium frying pan, heat the olive oil. Flavor the chicken breasts with salt and pepper. Cook the chicken breasts until cooked through (approximately 5 – 7 minutes each side).

2. Cook the pasta, as stated in the instruction of the package. Cook the snow peas with the pasta. Scoop 1 cup of the pasta water. Drain the pasta and peas, set aside.

3. Once the chicken is cooked, slice diagonally. Return back the chicken in the frying pan. Add the pasta

sauce. If the mixture seems dry, add some of the pasta water to the desired consistency. Heat, then divide into bowls. Serve immediately.

Nutrition:

Calories - 140

Protein - 34g

Carbohydrates - 52g

Fat - 17g

Sodium - 118mg

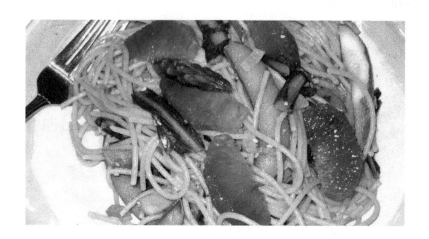

Chicken with Noodles

Preparation time: 15 minutes

Cooking time: 30 minutes

Servings: 6

Ingredients:

- 4 chicken breasts, skinless, boneless

- 1-pound pasta (angel hair, or linguine, or ramen)

- ½ teaspoon sesame oil

- 1 Tablespoon canola oil

- 2 Tablespoons chili paste

- 1 onion, diced

- 2 garlic cloves, chopped coarsely

- ½ cup of soy sauce

- ½ medium cabbage, sliced

- 2 carrots, chopped coarsely

Directions:

1. Cook your pasta in a large pot. Mix the canola oil, sesame oil, and chili paste and heat for 25 seconds in a large pot. Add the onion, cook for 2 minutes. Put the garlic and fry within 20 seconds. Add the

chicken, cook on each side 5 - 7 minutes, until cooked through.

2. Remove the mix from the pan, set aside. Add the cabbage, carrots, cook until the vegetables are tender. Pour everything back into the pan. Add the noodles. Pour in the soy sauce and combine thoroughly. Heat for 5 minutes. Serve immediately.

Nutrition:

Calories - 110

Protein - 30g

Carbohydrates - 32g

Sugars - 0.1g

Fat - 18g

Sodium - 121mg

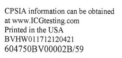